VERBAL MEDICINE

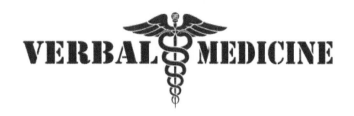

VERBAL MEDICINE

The Language of Healing™

MARC SACCO, RN, EMT-P, CRNH, BCH
&
ROGER WOODS, RN, CRNH, BCH, CI

TPW Publishing

ISBN: 9781795843560
www.patientwhisperers.com

Foreword

"Verbal Medicine" needs to be in the repertoire of every hypnotist -- both the book itself and the thought process it represents.   Marc Sacco and Roger Woods have provided us with a series of excellent examples and explanations of how careful semantics in medical situations and in hypnosis work can have amazing results.   They practice what they preach.

I was attending the wonderful lobster dinner which is the traditional ending to the National Guild of Hypnotists Annual Conference for our close knit group within the faculty. Just as one of our members was demonstrating a smoking cessation session on a restaurant patron, I got a very painful muscle spasm in my left leg. I knew that I might get it under control if I could stand up, but I was unable to, and was trying (badly) to stifle a horrendous scream.   Roger and Marc quickly surrounded me, and one of them began telling me that pressure under my nose would cause the spasm to stop. I've used pressure there to stop a sneeze -- many of us have. But I had never considered that location for anything else. As they spoke to me, the spasm came under control quite rapidly. After the pain subsided, I analyzed my case. I knew their mechanism had been Waking Hypnosis accompanied by pressure on a sensitive spot. I teach Waking Hypnosis and have used it for over 60 years. But I had never had it applied on me in a pain situation with such overwhelming speed and skill. They were positively amazing.

People who write interesting books are not uncommon. Those who not only do so, but superbly practice what they preach are persons who should be listened to and read!

—Col H. Larry Elman, USAF Ret'd, CH, CI

Mantra

Our Mantra at The Patient Whisperers™ is:

"Wouldn't you agree your brain controls every cell in your body right down to the chemical releases?"
(Wait for agreement)
"So why not make it work FOR you instead of AGAINST you?!"

— **TPW**

This is such a powerful convincer that we encourage everyone to memorize it and use it with everyone you speak to regarding Verbal Medicine™, Hypnosis, NLP, etc. **Everyone** agrees with the statement (who can argue with its logic) because it is a true fact that can't be disputed. It also gives them the internal permission to make change using their brain! Therefore, when you have agreement, you have compliance and when you have compliance, you have change.

CHAPTER ONE
Who in the HELL do we think WE are?!

Origins of The Patient Whisperers™

Before we learned the skill of hypnosis and NLP to enhance our practice, we were known in our emergency department as "Patient Whisperers." When there was a difficult patient or a psych patient stuck in the car out in the parking lot and they couldn't talk them in, our colleagues would come get one of us. If there was an irate patient in the hallway, again they would ask us to go talk to them because, for some reason when one of us talked to them, they calmed down and they willingly did what we needed them to do.

We had no idea that we were natural hypnotists before we became certified hypnotists. We just naturally had that language. As you read more and learn what we do, you may discover that you too are a natural hypnotist. We had that innate rapport and we had the right demeanor. So when we received our training by The National Guild of Hypnotists, Inc. at The New York Awareness Center with Mark Schwimmer, and we realized how important this could be to fundamentally changing the way we treat patients across the whole spectrum of healthcare, we thought to ourselves we have the perfect name. It's natural. We're going to brand this. We're going to be The Patient Whisperers™ and we're going to train other healthcare professionals not only to be hypnotists, we're going to train them in our methods, and in doing so they're going to be Patient Whisperers also. That is our mission and Verbal Medicine™ is our method. Because we are "working" nurses in an emergency department of a busy trauma center in the New England area our training is focused mainly on one of the most influential groups and frankly the group that has the most direct patient contact in the healthcare profession…Nurses. However, over the last 25 years in nursing schools the emphasis has been placed on teaching the science of nursing to the detriment of every patient nurses come in contact with, because the most important element of that care, the art of nursing, is missing.

That is why Verbal Medicine™ is the very essence of the art of nursing. That is the difference between a nurse and an exceptional caregiver/ healer. We all can remember that special person that made a difference at a time when it really mattered with a comforting word, soft touch, and a healing presence.

We invite you now to close your eyes for 1 minute and think of that person right now.

Did you visualize that special person that had an impact on your life at that time of need?

The Patient Whisperers believe that we as nurses can have that same reaction/response/memory and more importantly establish an Access Point™ for change that can last a lifetime. We believe (and have demonstrated successfully in our own Emergency Department) that fundamental change can be made by nurses who model the behaviors of The Patient Whisperers. Our colleagues who are nurses, doctors, and technicians have witnessed the amazing results we have and either request to get training from us, ask us to help with their difficult patients, or beg us to help them with their own problems… and we do all three!

After a while, we were getting so many requests from our friends, family, patients and staff members, that we began seeing them outside of work. Then people began reaching out to us when the word of our successes began to spread. When it became too much, we realized we needed to open our own clinic. Before long (actually after using Verbal Medicine™ on over 25,000 patients in under five years), we became Subject Matter Experts regarding Hypnosis in Healthcare and we started getting requests for speaking engagements to educate others in using our techniques, such as Verbal Medicine™ in the healthcare profession and Verbal SWAT™ in the EMS, Fire, and Police professions. And so, The Patient Whisperers opened offices in Connecticut and Vermont. Currently, they travel around lecturing internationally as Subject Matter Experts on Hypnosis in Healthcare (in their spare time!)

The Founders

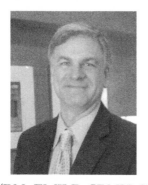

Marc Sacco (RN, EMT-P, CRNH, BCH, CEN) is a National Guild of Hypnotists Board Certified Consulting Hypnotist, NLP Practitioner, a Registered Nurse in the Emergency Department and Hospital Supervisor at Dartmouth-Hitchcock's Mt. Ascutney Hospital, a Board Certified Emergency Nurse, an Instructor holding several FEMA/Homeland Security certifications, and is one of the Founders of The Patient Whisperers in the Greater Danbury, CT area.

Mr. Sacco has held multiple roles in Emergency Management Services including Emergency Medical Technician, Paramedic, RN, Charge Nurse, Instructor, Supervisor, and Owner/Manager. Mr. Sacco was the recipient of the "Top Gun" award for finishing at the top of his class in both EMT and

Paramedic school. Marc holds a BA in Film and Theatre from Florida State University, AA from St. Petersburg College, AS (graduated with honors) in Nursing from Excelsior College and is a Board Certified Emergency Nurse.

Marc has been involved in Emergency Medicine for over 30 years, including over 23 years as a Paramedic and over 10 years as an Emergency Department Nurse.

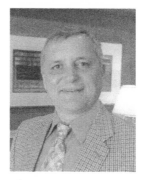

Roger Woods (RN, CRNH, BCH, CI) is a National Guild of Hypnotists Board Certified Consulting Hypnotist, NGH Certified Instructor of Hypnosis, NLP Practitioner, a Registered Nurse in the Emergency Department at Danbury Hospital's Level II Trauma Center, a FEMA/ Homeland Security Instructor holding several certifications in many areas of disaster preparedness/management, the 2016 national recipient of The Everyday Hero Award from the American Federation of Teachers, a college and high school healthcare professions instructor, and one of the Founders of The Patient Whisperers in the Greater Danbury, CT area.

Roger holds an Associates degree in Nursing and a Bachelors degree in Healthcare Administration with a concentration in Management.

Roger has held many roles throughout his nursing career including, Clinical Instructor, Emergency Department Charge Nurse, Private

Duty Nurse, Agency/Staff Relief Nurse, School Nurse, Occupational Health Nurse, Endoscopy and PACU Nurse. Member of the Connecticut DMAT responding to Domestic and International Disasters.

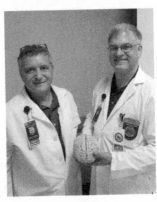

They are known as tireless advocates for their patients and are on a mission to enlighten both the medical world and their clients about the phenomenal advantages of integrating complementary medicine into the current practice of "modern" medicine.

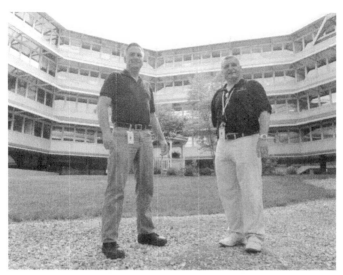

Together, they have created and developed several
groundbreaking programs to bring Mind / Body
Medicine into the mainstream including Verbal
Medicine™, Verbal SWAT™, VerbalDontics™,
VerbalRescue™, MyndBodyGym™, and the
CRNH™ nursing credential project.

Hypnosis

Many wonderful books have been written explaining what Hypnosis is and isn't and we will leave that up to you to research more information if you desire. A basic definition of Hypnosis is:

"A state or condition in which the subject becomes highly responsive to suggestions. The hypnotized individual seems to follow instructions in an uncritical, automatic fashion and attends closely only to those aspects of the environment made relevant by the hypnotist."[1]

Hypnosis is a system or collection of methods that enables one to bypass the critical factor of the conscious mind allowing direct access to the subconscious mind allowing mind and body to share information more effectively.

All Hypnosis is considered Self Hypnosis!

Neuro Linguistic Programming (NLP)

Many wonderful books have also been written explaining what Neuro Linguistic Programing (NLP) is and isn't and we will leave that up to you to research more information if you desire. A basic definition of NLP is:

Dr Richard Bandler invented the term "Neuro-Linguistic Programming" in the 1970s. He was recently asked to write the definition of Neuro-Linguistic Programming that appears in the Oxford English Dictionary. It says:

Neuro-Linguistic Programming: "a model of interpersonal communication chiefly concerned with the relationship between successful patterns of behaviour and the subjective experiences (esp. patterns of thought) underlying them" and "a system of alternative therapy based on this which seeks to educate people in self-awareness and effective communication, and to change their patterns of mental and emotional behaviour."[2]

What is Verbal Medicine™?

Verbal Medicine™ is the language of healing. It is
the positive communication between the mind, the
body and the spirit. It is the best practice of the
integration of healthcare, hypnosis and NLP. By
using the inherent influence that people are giving
healthcare   professionals,   Verbal   Medicine™
enhances   the   suggestions   made   to   become
powerful   healing   words.   All   healthcare
professionals have this influence of healing as our
patients are highly receptive to suggestions, and
we need to watch what we say because each and
every word we use can either help or hinder the
patient's response and recovery. For example, let's
talk about the PAIN Scale! We are accustomed to
ask our patients, "How much PAIN are you in?
What is your PAIN level? On a scale of 0 to 10 with
10 being the worst pain you ever experienced and
zero being no PAIN at all, what is your PAIN
number?" instead we use the following, "How
comfortable are you right now? What is your
comfort level" With zero being very comfortable
and 10 being very uncomfortable, what number
describes your comfort level right now?" Do you

see a difference? Do you hear a change? Does that feel better to you? So, we suggest, every Healthcare professional needs to memorize our mantra (on the first page) and use it as a powerful convincer! Verbal Medicine™ fundamentally shifts how we as Healthcare Professionals provide care by changing the perception, reaction, and results of our patient's experience while enhancing and rejuvenating the provider. Verbal Medicine™ changes what we say, how we say things, and when we say things to elicit positive results and become Better at the Bedside™. It creates, within the healthcare professional, a chain of influence that allows them to drive the care. Using a unique combination of nursing, hypnosis, NLP (Neuro Linguistic Programming), and healing touch, we are able to achieve amazing results, instant rapport, better compliance, faster recovery, and more satisfied patients on a consistent basis within a busy New England Level II Trauma Center Emergency Department. We have used Verbal Medicine™ on over 25,000 patients in less than five years! We have honed our skills and distilled our techniques into a very efficient and successful method known as Verbal Medicine™. In that time we have also seen a fundamental shift in how other healthcare providers view hypnosis and NLP (in the form of Verbal Medicine™) and how they have began to consider it as an important tool to be used daily alongside more traditional treatments. Having witnessed the positive results time and time again, they have accepted it as an integrated part of our nursing process and actively sought out our services for their patients! In addition, many of our fellow nurses approached us to teach them how to do Verbal Medicine™ as well. Thus was born the CRNH™ project. (More about that at the end of the book)

Why Verbal Medicine™ should be used

Because everything that is said by a healthcare professional to the patient has so much weight that every little word can have dramatic consequences (for better or for worse!) in the delivery of care so… take care in the delivery.

It is summed up in one of the foundational quotes that we have based The Patient Whisperers™ on…

"You will relieve, more effectually, unreasonable suffering from reasonable causes by giving him something new to think of or to look at than by all the logic in the world."
—Florence Nightingale[3]

So Verbal Medicine™ (we'll call it "VMed") is an acute awareness that everything that is spoken to and received by someone at a pivotal moment which we call an "Access Point" can either heal or hinder their care. Everyone who is experiencing an intense event (such as an emergency) is already in a light to medium trance due to the focusing nature of the event. They are already highly suggestible if you have the knowledge to identify the Access Points. VMed is that knowledge! You can dynamically shift their recovery in the blink of an eye it's that quick!

In traditional Hypnosis the pretalk is very important. As a matter of fact, in our clinical practice we spend an hour (or more) in the 2 hour initial session just doing pretalk! In the Emergency Department (we'll call it the "ED") we didn't have the luxury of having that time so we needed to develop an efficient and effective way of accomplishing our goal. Our efforts led to the development of VMed and Access Points. In many of the traditional techniques of hypnosis and NLP, we identify the Initial Sensitizing Event (ISE) as the start of a particular problem and work up from there. In the Emergency Setting, people are so focused on their current issue that it overwhelms their mind. This became our moment to make the right connection and make change happen. This was the Access Point! When accessed properly it can open the patient to dynamic changes immediately! Also, as we have witnessed many times, when providers don't recognize these Access Points they can either pass right by them (like an exit on the highway) missing the perfect opportunity to help their patients heal quickly or even worse they stumble "off the exit" into an Access Point and say the absolute wrong thing that sets their patient up for failure, relapse, or even death! (Not that they intended to do harm, they just don't know what to say!) One of our favorite (and most powerful) quotes is:

"Words are, of course, the most powerful drug used by mankind."

— Rudyard Kipling

The Harvard Studies

(Excerpts from Harvard Magazine)[4]

TWO WEEKS INTO Ted Kaptchuk's first randomized clinical drug trial, nearly a third of his 270 subjects complained of awful side effects. All the patients had joined the study hoping to alleviate severe arm pain: carpal tunnel, tendinitis, chronic pain in the elbow, shoulder, wrist. In one part of the study, half the subjects received pain-reducing pills; the others were offered acupuncture treatments. And in both cases, people began to call in, saying they couldn't get out of bed. The pills were making them sluggish, the needles caused swelling and redness; some patients' pain ballooned to nightmarish levels. "The side effects were simply amazing," Kaptchuk explains; curiously, they were exactly what patients had been warned their treatment might produce. But even more astounding, most of the other patients reported real relief, and those who received acupuncture felt even better than those on the anti-pain pill. These were exceptional findings: no one had ever proven that acupuncture worked better than painkillers. But Kaptchuk's study didn't prove it, either. The pills his team had given patients were actually made of cornstarch; the "acupuncture" needles were retractable shams that never pierced the skin. The study wasn't aimed at comparing two treatments. It was designed to compare two fakes.

But researchers have found that placebo treatments—interventions with no active drug ingredients—can stimulate real physiological responses, from changes in heart rate and blood pressure to chemical activity in the brain, in cases involving pain, depression, anxiety, fatigue, and even some symptoms of Parkinson's.

The challenge now, says Kaptchuk, is to uncover the mechanisms behind these physiological responses—what is happening in our bodies, in our brains, in the method of placebo delivery (pill or needle, for example), even in the room where placebo treatments are administered (are the physical surroundings calming? is the doctor caring or curt?). The placebo effect is actually many effects woven together—some stronger than others —and that's what Kaptchuk hopes his "pill versus needle" study shows. The experiment, among the first to tease apart the components of placebo response, shows that the methods of placebo administration are as important as the administration itself, he explains. It's valuable insight for any caregiver: patients' perceptions matter, and the ways healthcare providers frame perceptions can have significant effects on their patients' health.

But years of considering the question led him to his next clinical experiment: What if he simply told people they were taking placebos? The question ultimately inspired a pilot study, published by the peer-reviewed science and medicine journal PLOS ONE in 2010, that yielded his most famous findings to date. His team again compared two groups of IBS sufferers. One group received no treatment. The other patients were told they'd be taking fake, inert drugs (delivered in bottles labeled "placebo pills") and told also that placebos often have healing effects.

The study's results shocked the investigators themselves: even patients who knew they were taking placebos described real improvement, reporting twice as much symptom relief as the no-treatment group. That's a difference so significant, says Kaptchuk, it's comparable to the improvement seen in trials for the best real IBS drugs.

The first evidence of a physiological basis for the placebo effect appeared in the late 1970s, when researchers studying dental patients found that by chemically blocking the release of endorphins—the brain's natural pain relievers—scientists could also block the placebo effect. This suggested that placebo treatments spurred chemical responses in the brain that are similar to those of active drugs, a theory borne out two decades later by brain-scan technology. Researchers like neuroscientist Fabrizio Benedetti at the University of Turin have since shown that many neurotransmitters are at work— including chemicals that use the same pathways as opium and marijuana. Studies by other researchers have shown that placebos increase dopamine (a chemical that affects emotions and sensations of pleasure and reward) in the brains of Parkinson's patients, and patients suffering from depression who've been given placebos reveal changes in electrical and metabolic activity in several different regions of the brain.

Kaptchuk and his team have begun to take steps in that direction, continuing to ask new questions and push the boundaries of placebo research. A study published online this past year in the Proceedings of the National Academy of Sciences demonstrated that the placebo response can occur even at the unconscious level. The team showed that images flashed on a screen for a fraction of a second—too quickly for conscious recognition—could trigger the response,but only if patients had learned earlier to associate those specific images with healing. Thus, when patients enter a room containing medical equipment they associate with the possibility of feeling better, "the mind may automatically make associations that lead to actual positive health outcomes," says psychiatry research fellow Karin Jensen, the study's lead author.[5]

Where can Verbal Medicine™ be used?

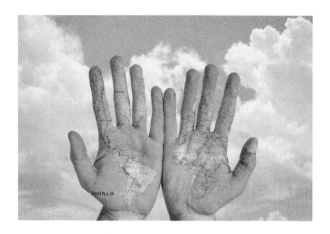

While VMed was developed in the Emergency setting for healthcare professionals, it can really be used anywhere in any situation! By learning to identify Access Points and the languaging techniques within VMed, you can apply this to many different things in your life. We use it daily in everything we do!

Here are a few places we have used it…

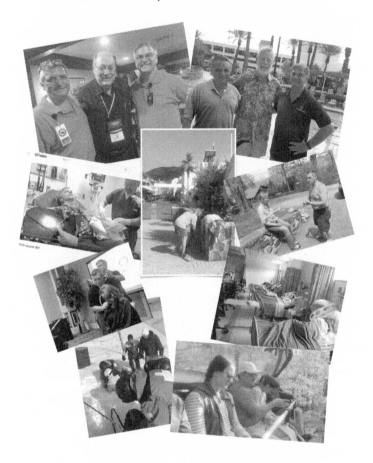

Boats, chairlifts, ambulances, restaurants, pools, bridges, cat scans, subways, trains, planes, supermarkets, football games, hotels, seminars/ conferences, classrooms, roadsides, ski resorts…

When can Verbal Medicine™ be used?

Ready? ……. Wait for it……..Anytime!

Seriously, we truly use this anytime it is needed! Whether it is at work in the emergency department or in the islands on vacation, we use it whenever it is needed! It has not only become a natural part of our nursing process but also an integral part of our life. What more can we say!

Who needs to use Verbal Medicine™?

Even though the foundation of VMed was built for healthcare workers, we have adapted it to meet other needs and situations. It quite seamlessly has been used in Healthcare settings (Verbal Medicine™), Emergency Medicine (Verbal SWAT™), Dental offices (VerbalDontics™), and Fitness Centers (MyndBodyGym™) as well as in our daily lives (Verbal Rescue™). It should be used by everyone to experience their world in a better way and enhance their interactions with the world around them!

How do we use it?

How can we possibly use this in the chaotic environment of a busy Emergency Department!? Unlike traditional hypnosis where you typically go to an office with the room darkened, soothing music playing, and a nice comfy chair; we are forced to deal with noise, lighting, activity, and a patient that isn't in a calm state! We needed to develop methods that worked for us in that environment and that worked quickly. As Bruce Lee once said, "Absorb what is useful, Discard what is not, Add what is uniquely your own" and, "Use only that which works, and take it from any place you can find it." So we looked at everything and played with many techniques from many different sources from hypnosis, NLP, nursing, theatre, construction, painting, parenting, and basically anything from our life experiences!

We use it as an integrated part of our nursing process. At this point, we cannot separate it from our nursing. We have increased our awareness of what we should be doing and saying as well as what is being said and done around us. All of which can be an tremendous asset or a disastrous detriment! That brings us to another critical part of Verbal Medicine, Utilization. We use everything around us to enhance the care of our patients. It is an essential part of the Verbal Medicine process that cannot be overstated. (See the chapter on Utilization for a great example)

CHAPTER TWO

Foundations and Theory

Foundations and Theory

Our foundation in healthcare was broken. Healthcare started out with the noble purpose of providing care to the sick and injured. Then came a seismic shift when healthcare went from focusing on being a "service to the patient" to being a "fee for service." As it became a profitable business and the focus began pointing away from the patient and onto the profits, it attracted people from other industries who felt they could run healthcare like any other industry. Instead of getting to the heart of the matter, they didn't realize it was a matter of the heart. While appearances may have been kept up, the business model has clearly favored the drive towards doing more with less and it has resulted in a dramatic decrease in patient satisfaction and an increase in staff burnout and dissatisfaction. That was where we were... our foundations were personally crumbling and broken. We needed to find a way to fix it or we were not going to last much longer! We were both ready to leave the profession. We were "burnt to a crisp!" There was an imbalance of energy. More energy was going out than we were taking in and most of the energy available seemed to be negative all around us. Something needed to change....soon!

And then there was an opportunity for change! Not some magical bolt of lightning but through the perseverance of Roger who spent three years hounding the hospital foundation to give him a grant to get some training in hypnosis. It couldn't have come at a better time! From the moment we sat in that very first hypnosis training class and realized how essential this could be in changing the very foundations of our profession, we became filled with boundless positive energy! We have a simple statement written on our cards that says, " Relax, Renew, Rejuvenate, Re-Emerge, and Re-Engage" and it speaks volumes. In its very essence of simplicity, it states our core experience and while it is meant for everyone to embrace, it is, in fact, our origin...our story...our journey...and our rebirth. It points back to that seminal moment when we sat in that class realizing our world just fundamentally changed and that we now had the keys to drive our own success. We also knew we had a duty to change healthcare as we knew it...

Our beginnings in the basic training of hypnosis spurred us on to learn more techniques from many different masters such as Dave Elman, Milton Erickson, and Harry Arons. As we learned more, we experimented with blending these techniques with the nursing process and added even more skills using NLP (Neuro Linguistic Programming) all the while developing our own style by distilling the essentials from each discipline down to the most efficient methods. This was born out of the unique needs of a busy Level II Trauma Center's Emergency Department and became the early foundation of Verbal Medicine™.

The following are some of the core studies and abstracts that we have used to build the foundations of Verbal Medicine.

The Utah Study[6]

Abstract Background:

Medical management of acute pain among hospital inpatients may be enhanced by mind-body interventions.

Objective:

We hypothesized that a single, scripted session of mindfulness training focused on acceptance of pain or hypnotic suggestion focused on changing pain sensations through imagery would significantly reduce acute pain intensity and unpleasantness compared to a psychoeducation pain coping control. We also hypothesized that mindfulness and suggestion would produce significant improvements in secondary outcomes including relaxation, pleasant body sensations, anxiety, and desire for opioids, compared to the control condition.

Methods:

This three-arm, parallel-group randomized controlled trial conducted at a university-based hospital examined the acute effects of 15-min psychosocial interventions (mindfulness, hypnotic suggestion, psychoeducation) on adult inpatients reporting "intolerable pain" or "inadequate pain control." Participants ($N = 244$) were assigned to one of three intervention conditions: mindfulness ($n = 86$), suggestion ($n = 73$), or psychoeducation ($n = 85$).

Key Results:

Participants in the mind-body interventions reported significantly lower baseline-adjusted pain intensity post-intervention than those assigned to psychoeducation ($p < 0.001$, percentage pain reduction: mindfulness = 23%, suggestion = 29%, education = 9%), and lower baseline-adjusted pain unpleasantness ($p < 0.001$). Intervention conditions differed significantly with regard to relaxation ($p < 0.001$), pleasurable body sensations ($p = 0.001$), and desire for opioids ($p = 0.015$), but all three interventions were associated with a significant reduction in anxiety ($p < 0.001$).

Conclusions:

Brief, single-session mind-body interventions delivered by hospital social workers led to clinically significant improvements in pain and related outcomes, suggesting that such interventions may be useful adjuncts to medical pain management.

The Kansas Experiment

The Kansas Experiment sadly, the original data from this ground breaking study has been lost but a great account of it has been *preserved in the book "The Worst is Over"[7]. The following is an excerpt from a discussion with one of the authors:

"In the 1970s, psychiatrist M. Erik Wright created a pilot study on the effect of the right words on recovery, as described in Patient Communication for First Responders and EMS Personnel: The First Hour of Trauma by Donald Trent Jacobs, PhD. In what was called "The Kansas Experiment," Wright divided first responders into two groups. One utilized its customary mode of performance. The other followed these three steps set out by Wright:

Minimize extraneous input. Move the victim away from distractions, such as hysterical relatives and those who might offer dire prognoses or ask such damaging questions such as, "Is he going to die?"

Communicate this simple paragraph, word for word:

"The worst is over. We are taking you to the hospital. Everything is being made ready. Let your body concentrate on repairing itself and feeling secure. Let your heart, your blood vessels, everything, bring themselves into a state of preserving your life. Bleed just enough so as to cleanse the wound, and let the blood vessels close down so that your life is preserved. Your body weight, your body heat, everything, is being maintained. Things are being made ready in the hospital for you. We're getting there as quickly and safely as possible. You are now in a safe position. The worst is over."

Eliminate unrelated conversation. The program was all about the words, what was and wasn't said, during an emergency. His protocol required only the recitation of the paragraph above.

The results of the study were decisive. Patients who were in serious danger or were not expected to recover, but to whom this paragraph was said, surprised the first responders and emergency room physicians by doing much better than expected. Wright reported the only downside was the difficulty for the group of first responders using the protocol not to spoil the experiment by telling the others to try it, too.

While it is not necessarily recommended that you memorize the paragraph, it does succinctly demonstrate the protocol. Establish rapport. Reassure, but be realistic. Make therapeutic/ healing suggestions, and continue the rapport and sense of safety."

*(This information contained in The Worst is Over was given to them by Dr. Don "Four Arrows" Jacobs, author of many great books on Mind Body connections[8]. Four Arrows has become a friend and supporter of The Patient Whisperers and has not only given us access and permission to use his resources, but (as have the authors of The Worst is Over) has given us his support to replicate The Kansas Experiment in the future!

One of the important documents we base our nursing practice on is **Nursing as a Framework for Alternative/Complementary Modalities** We encourage you to look it up and download a copy of it to show you how Verbal Medicine (as well as other complementary modalities) can be used within the Nursing process. Early in our careers as Nurse Hypnotists we experienced some management push back from one of our "less educated, more narrow minded managers" and we researched how hypnosis and NLP fit under the nursing scope of practice and found this excellent abstract. The following is an excerpt from the abstract:

With nationwide interest in complementary healthcare, nurses have actively incorporated alternative/integrative modalities into their practice. Registered Nurses regularly attend continuing educational sessions on techniques such as acupressure, guided imagery, humor, massage, meditation, and therapeutic touch/healing touch. Review of continuing educational offerings advertised in holistic nursing newsletters and websites indicates that many nurses learn these techniques in sessions alongside other healthcare providers and are taught by non-nurses. In such situations, nurses may raise questions related to their legal scope of practice and the use of alternative/complementary modalities within professional nursing. When these techniques are taught by and practiced by individuals who are not nurses as well as by nurses, questions such as, "May a nurse practice guided imagery as an RN?", "May a nurse perform simple massage or therapeutic massage?" and "May a nurse practice therapeutic touch(TT) as a private, independent professional?" become critically important and not easily answered. While the practice of nursing is regulated by each state, ability to bring alternative/complementary modalities into a nursing context assists in defining the practice as part of professional nursing. When operating from a nursing perspective, nurses recognize that the ability to perform and use these techniques can be greatly enhanced when they integrate these techniques into the context of professional nursing. The purposes of this paper are to explore how a professional nursing context provides a discipline-specific direction to the practice of complementary/alternative modalities by adding qualities of assessment, reflection, and holism to the performance of the techniques, and to provide examples for nurses to incorporate alternative/complementary practices into care that is clearly identified as professional nursing. Noreen Cavan Frisch, PhD, RN, FAAN[9]

Another important document we refer to frequently and base our practice decisions on is The Joint Commission's R3 report[10] that outlines new requirements (former recommendations) to include non-pharmocologic treatment strategies for pain. Here are a few relevant sections paraphrased here (see footnotes for link to full article)

Requirement:

EP 2: The hospital provides nonpharmacologic pain treatment modalities.

Rationale:

While evidence for some nonpharmacologic modalities is mixed and/or limited, they may serve as a complementary approach for pain management and potentially reduce the need for opioid medications in some circumstances. The hospital should promote nonpharmacologic modalities by ensuring that patient preferences are discussed and, at a minimum, providing some nonpharmacologic treatment options relevant to their patient population. When a patient's preference for a safe nonpharmacologic therapy cannot be provided, hospitals should educate the patient on where the treatment may be accessed post-discharge. **Nonpharmacologic strategies**

include, but are not limited to: physical modalities (for example, acupuncture therapy, chiropractic therapy, osteopathic manipulative treatment, massage therapy, and physical therapy), **relaxation therapy**, and cognitive behavioral therapy.

Requirement:

EP 3: The hospital treats the patient's pain or refers the patient for treatment. Note: Treatment strategies for pain may include nonpharmacologic, pharmacologic, or a combination of approaches.

Rationale:

Referrals may be required for patients who present with complex pain management needs, such as the opioid-addicted patient, the patient who is at high risk for adverse events and who requires treatment with opioids, or a patient whose pain management needs exceed the expertise of the patient's attending licensed independent practitioner.

CHAPTER THREE
Tools: Utilization

Utilization
The Essence of Verbal Medicine

Verbal Medicine uses many approaches and modalities gleaned from the healing arts, complementary medicine including Hypnosis and NLP combined with the nursing process.

The Patient Whisperers have taken the best of the best techniques and have condensed them into a working format that leans heavily on Milton Erickson's theory of having the ability to utilize anything and everything about a patient to help them change, including their beliefs, words that they use, cultural background, personal habits and anything and everything else of use. The Patient Whisperers go one step further in using every sound and sensation while engaged in the change process. It doesn't matter if it's loud, quiet, bright, dark, hot or cold, it doesn't matter if it's the night time or the daytime, summer or winter, in fact all surrounding sensations are welcomed and used to bring the subject into a deep trance by convincing the subconscious mind that all of the sensations are real. And if the sensations are perceived as being real, then all the suggestions you impart are just as real. Right?

"All Aboard"

(As related by Roger)

On one occasion I had an evening appointment that was running late, by the time the client arrived it was close to 6:30 PM, after the pre-talk it was close to 7:15pm before we entered into a progressive relaxation for the session. The office was all set, the lights were low, the background music was soothing, it was a perfect setting for relaxation and we began. Fifteen minutes into the session somewhere off in the distance I heard a sound, a kind of muffled clinking/banging sound. It was a sound that I had identified sometime before, it was the vacuum the office cleaners used on the tile floors in the hallways. And it reminded me of a train traveling down the tracks. However tonight, instead of the sound remaining off in the distance, I noticed it was moving towards the office, I came to the realization the office cleaner was headed my way and with each second the sound of the vacuum on the tile floor was increasing with volume. As I continued with this session, I came to the conclusion that he was definitely coming our way and there was no way to avoid the noise. So, I immediately switched my session and decided to utilize this new development and use it to enhance my clients experience. It sounds like a train coming down the hallway......and so it is. I thought to myself, trains pick items up at the station and take them away to faraway places, right? So I began;

"In a moment I want you to imagine you are at a train station and I want you to visualize putting all of those problems, issues, memories and worries that were holding you back from success on that train, in fact, you are going to place all of those useless items in a large suitcase and seal it, or lock it, or weld it shut so that it cannot open. Everyone of these useless items in that suitcase were preventing you from going forward, right? You know, there was a time long ago where those items were useful and now they are not. Now they need to go far away as you have no use of them anymore, right? So send them away on the train that you hear coming down the track. (At this time the noise outside the office has begun to get even louder!) So I continue, " Now get ready to put that suitcase on the train and allow it to go away right now... far, far away as you have no use of those things anymore, those things that had been holding you back from your success."

And then all of a sudden it stopped. That noise outside the office had stopped and a few seconds later the door to the office began to open slowly. And I'm greeted by the smiling face of the office cleaner as he peered in from the hallway! Immediately, I put my hand in a stop gesture to prevent him from talking but it was in vain as he asked "Can I get the garbage?". (What!!! That's perfect, I'll use it) "Yes...", I began, as he finished emptying the garbage pail and started to leave, I added, "...take that garbage away, we have no need of it anymore!"

To my amazement, my client did not stir one bit! So deep in trance was she that this interaction did not disturb her relaxation state at all.

As the door was almost completely closed, I said, "ALL ABOARD!...put your baggage and garbage on the train for a destination far, far away."

And then, as if right on cue, the vacuuming started again and I heard the cleaner making his way further down the hall and fading off into the distance as I repeat twice more the statement about placing the baggage on the train for a far far away destination. Finally, silence falls and I finish the session and I bring her out of trance. A few moments later, she said that the session was amazing claiming that she actually felt as if she was at the train station and felt the train coming down the tracks, and even heard the conductor saying "All aboard!", and excitedly exclaiming, "It felt so real!"

The lesson here is that by utilizing everything in your domain you are providing powerful convincers to your suggestions, and if it begins to feel real, then it is real, right? Always remember..."Reality isn't real! Its our perception of reality that is real to us!" Therefore, if you can change your perception, you can make change to your reality!" (Disclaimer: all the laws of physics are still currently in effect so please don't try to walk through walls or fly without a plane etc.!!!)

CHAPTER FOUR

Tools: Healing Breathes and Relaxation

One of the simplest and most effective tools we use is the "Healing Breath/Relaxation" induction. We have incorporated it into our nursing process as a natural way of building a trust and rapport with our patient. It allows us to give the patient an immediate gift of relaxation which then sets them up for a successful visit. It also serves as a convincer that we can build greater results from! Everyone breathes.....most do it wrong on a daily basis! Most people breath shallow using their upper chest and shoulders to take air into the upper lobes of their lungs. When we teach them the "Healing Breaths" they learn to do a deeper "Belly Breath" using their diaphragms and getting the air into the lower lobes. This has several physiological benefits that allow the patient to naturally relax.

First, it gives their body more oxygen to use which in turn replenishes their muscles, organs, and brains. This lets their body work less at getting what it needs thus relaxing the body. Second, the diaphragm movement helps stimulate the vagus nerve which slows the heart rate, respirations, and releases chemicals to calm and relax the body and mind.

The Patient Whisperers'
Healing Breath/Relaxation Script

Relax, Renew, Rejuvenate, Re-emerge, and Re-engage

("….." after each word indicates a pause)

In a moment....

you will begin three healing....relaxing breaths.... In through the nose for 3 seconds, hold it in for 3 seconds and exhale out through the mouth for 6 seconds…

Now....let's get into a comfortable position before you begin....

and notice...sometime between the first breath and the third breath....

Just allowing.... yourself.... to close your eyes....

notice   and   experience   each   breath.... in....and....out

as you begin.... to relax....

So allow your busy mind and tension filled body.... to have the opportunity to relax....together. That's right....

Now....as your eyes are closed....

allow your healing breaths to guide you.... deeper....into....relaxation....

Allow each....breath.... you inhale through the nose.... to inhale calmness....

And with each exhale out through the mouth.... remove and release....stress....and tension....becoming loose and limp....and just letting go.... that's right....

Now....

Focus on both of your eyes....and the area around them, that's right....

Begin to allow all the tiny muscles around your eyes....to....relax....that's right....Now....

Allow all the energy....to evaporate....to dissipate.... relaxing....and releasing....and letting go....

To the point....where those eye lids are so....so.... relaxed....so loose....so heavy.....and so relaxed....

That....even if you try, try, try....you wouldn't, nor couldn't....open your eyes.........that's right, now stop..trying....that's right.

Just allow them to be completely....loose and limp....that's right....relaxing and.....releasing

Now....allow that wonderful relaxation....that you have right now....to move....to the top of your head....

Right....now allow that wonderful relaxation....to move and soothe out....all the tension in the small muscles of the scalp....that's right....

Slow....and deeply....those areas of tension are becoming.... less and less.... becoming loose and limp....and sooooo relaxed.....right....

Now....allow your wonderful relaxation....to move and smooth those areas of tension in the side of your head....around the ears....moving down now....down into the jaw....relaxing and releasing the whole jaw now....and you may notice the relaxing of your throat...right....

Now....send that relaxation to the side of your neck.... to the back of your neck....and down....down....down to your shoulders ....that's right....

Those shoulders....that hold all of the tension of the day....the week....the month.....the year....

Imagine now.... your relaxation begins to dissolve that tension....little by little at first....relaxing.... and releasing.... tension....

Imagine   that   tension   dissolving....
evaporating....dissipating....as the shoulders begin
to   loosen....releasing....relaxing....becoming   loose
and limp....and letting go....yes....that's right....

Now....send   that   sensation....your
relaxation....down.... down....your arms to your
e l b o w s . . . . d o w n   t o   t h e
forearms....wrists....hands....fingers....and   all   the
way to the tips of the nails....that's right

Right now....send that relaxation.... that you have
created to the chest....

Allow the chest muscles to relax.... with every
b r e a t h . . . . r e l a x i n g . . . . r e l e a s i n g . . . . a n y
tension....becoming   loose....   and   limp....and   so
relaxed....that's right.....

Allowing that sensation....your relaxation....now,
to move into your belly

Relaxing those abdominal muscles....

Relaxing all of your spine, from the top all the
way down to the bottom.... relaxing....releasing and
letting go....that's right.

Relaxing and releasing the muscles....of the
pelvis/hips

Going   down....down....down,   relaxing....and
releasing....and letting go....that's right

Now,   send   that   relaxation
down....down....down....

Into the thigh muscles....allowing all of that
tension.... to dissipate....evaporate....release and
relax....that's right

Now.... send your relaxation to the
knees....down....down.... down, to the calves and
shins....moving down into your ankles.... heels....
and the soles of your feet.... all the way to the tips
of your toes, that's right....that's right....

Now....you are so deeply relaxed....so deeply
relaxed from the top of your head to the tips of
your toes....Relaxing....releasing....and letting go....

Now.... anytime you need that wonderful
relaxation....all you need to do, is visualize this
relaxation.... and remember the path you followed
to get here.... enabling you to remember and feel
this deep relaxation again.

And anytime.... anytime....you close your eyes
and take those three healing breaths....you will find
your way back to this wonderful....deep relaxation.

Now...take 5, 10 or 15 minutes to enjoy your
wonderful relaxation....

Take this time now.... to refocus on what you
want....what you need.... from your life right

now....and focus right now.... on what you need to do to get it.....

And imagine yourself right now.... having what it is you need from your life right now....

Allow yourself to love and be loved.....Become the healer.... and heal yourself and in turn you will heal others through your actions....your thoughts ....and your wise words....

And be successful.... by seeing yourself successful each and every time you close your eyes.... and take those three.... healing breaths so you can return time after time, quicker and deeper each time to this wonderful state of relaxation.... because when you see it....you can act it.... and you can be it....right

Knowing that there are no longer any mistakes in your life....just lessons that you have learned....learn from them....and teach those lessons to others what you have learned about yourself....

Life lessons are made to share. So share your lessons....

So choose a life to live.... choose to live life.... that is bigger....brighter....more loving and giving than the day before....

The future is not an upgrade on the present....
but an invitation to think in an entirely new way....
act in an entirely new way....and see and feel results
in an entirely new way....

And anytime you hear these words you will
instantly come back to the state of relaxation...

quicker.... deeper....each and every time.

And   when   you   feel....   Renewed....and
Rejuvenated....and you are ready....Re-emerge and
.... Simply.... Re-engage.... That's right.

Here is a sample script from one of our good friends and mentors Captain M. Ron Eslinger[11]...

Relaxing Breath Script

This should be taught to every client and used as an anchor between sessions – great to teach as a takeaway when you do a talk for service organizations

Ask the client to take a very deep breath. After they let it out have them notice how they stiffened up their chest, their neck and many will bite down clinching their jaw and not be aware of it.

Next tell them to just gently push out their stomach and notice how they automatically suck air into their lungs. The reason for this is the negative pressure created when they push out their stomach. The diaphragm drops down creating a negative pressure in the chest, which automatically expands the lungs, sucking in air.

Explain that the lungs have five lobes and that when many people take a very deep breath they expand the two upper lobes of the lungs much more than the lower lobes. Let them know that the two lower lobes of the lungs have more blood vessels and more Alveoli (air sacks); therefore more oxygen gets from the lungs to the tissues.

Oxygen is relaxing and healing and allows a major decrease in stress.

It is also important to explain that the Vagus nerve runs through the diaphragm. And when the diaphragm is hyper stretched it activates the Vagus nerve which stimulate anti-stress hormones.

So by taking an abdominal breath at least once an hour, it changes the stress response.

The best way to do this is to breathe in for a count of three, hold the breath three counts and breathe out for six counts and to do that hourly. Also find some time in the day when they can take ten breaths in that manner. This type of breathing is a major component of a client's success.

CHAPTER FIVE

Tools: Rapport and Body Language

Rapport and Body Language
Look who's talking

Verbal Medicine™ was developed to enhance communication between the healthcare giver and the patient and uses both forms of language to communicate. Both the spoken and unspoken. Problems and issues in everyday communication arise when what is spoken is not matched with the bodies own unique language. We all have had experience with this. Something tells you (your subconscious) what the person is saying may not be true or misleading. There is no congruence between the spoken word and body language. It might be the way they hold their head, the tone of their voice, the speed of delivery, the shifting of the eyes, the touching of the nose, the hiding of the mouth and hands. You just can't put your finger on it, but your subconscious mind is paying attention. The more you become attuned to body language and decipher it's code, the easier it becomes to build rapport and compliance. Knowing what to say is important, knowing how and when to say it is a skill worth learning. Over the years Verbal Medicine™ has been tested on over 25,000 patients, every single one had some Verbal Medicine™ component to their care. And every single one of those patients benefited one way or another from Verbal Medicine™, that was cost-effective, time efficient and came with no detrimental side effects.

Finding the Energy to Heal.

(As related by Roger)

One night I stayed to work a double in the Emergency Department. By doing this, my shift changed from 10 hours to 18 hours. A practice I have been doing at least once, if not twice a week. This time I was ending a week that I had worked three. Anyway, I had just finished working a full 10 hours with no break and was taking another assignment for the upcoming eight hours overnight. I was assigned observation, which is the behavioral health area serving patients requiring a psych evaluation and can run the spectrum of mental and behavioral issues. We also cater to well known local drunks, who are found by police intoxicated on public streets, and everything in between. It's a great place to work and play with language skills.

Within 30 minutes of starting the midnight to 8 am shift, the night manager of the emergency department, came over to where I was working and stated she had a special request for me. It seemed that one of our techs/nursing assistants was threatening to go home due to pain in her leg because of sciatic nerve pain running down the whole of one of her legs. Given that we would be working short staffed if she did indeed leave the department, the night manager thought I could help her out with some techniques so she would stay. Now, the night manager knew that I was skilled in changing people's perception of pain and she asked if I would work with the tech who was threatening to leave. I listened to the manager explain she needed to keep the tech at work as they were very short-staffed at night and if she did go home it would impact heavily on the whole department. I was on board until she mentioned the person's name. Having worked with this person previously many times, I didn't have a good rapport with her and didn't feel I had the right energy required to work with her. She had always been a very negative person and did not have good energy. You know, that one person who as soon as they enter the room all the life is sucked out of it. Well, this was that kind of tech. As you know in life, you have certain people that you instantly click with and those that you don't. Well, this one I didn't.

I instantly said no, and gave the charge nurse the reason why, I didn't feel the energy and I didn't want to use any of my energy to help her, feeling that she didn't deserve it. (Energy goes to where energy flows.) After all, I was tired and I still had seven hours to go. So, as soon as I made that statement to the night manager she left my area.

It turned out that the tech didn't leave and was trying to work through the pain. An hour or two went by and I had to leave my area to go talk to a doctor regarding a patient requiring some medication. I proceeded to the area where the doctors sit to write orders and hung out there for around five minutes before I began to feel a "disturbance in the force". Literally, I felt energy, I felt a presence, it was behind me. I didn't have to look behind me to know who it was. I knew it was the tech, as I turned around I confirmed my own suspicions. We looked at each other and instantly we had rapport because I knew she was ready to work on her pain. And so… was I. She looked pale, sad, and her posture was hunched over.

I directed her to one of the trauma rooms, I told her to lie on the stretcher and get herself comfortable, in the meantime I dimmed the lights all the way down and closed the glass doors sealing the room from loud noises. I instructed her to take three healing breaths and then began a progressive relaxation, and soon she was in a wonderful, deep trance.

It was a quick 15 minute session. She went quick in to trance because she wanted this so badly. She had already convinced herself way before we started because she had seen our work with other coworkers and patients. I found out later she personally asked the night manager to ask me to help her. During this session, we simply changed her perception of the pain and gave her the control to dial it down, changed the shape and size and more importantly the intensity of the discomfort. I always use the word "allow" as this gives the control to the patient, it also gives them the responsibility and permission to go into trance. And as for me, we had rapport because my intent had changed, the energy in me was fired up because her energy was true, and even though I gave, I also received. This is a "do with" process and we can always get something out of it...if we choose.

I ended the session by giving her the gift of the three healing breaths and instructing her that she could use it anytime, anyplace and anywhere. She emerged from trance with a big smile on her face, her whole body had changed and her stance was upright and strong. Her skin was pink and glowing and she was smiling like a Cheshire cat. Her whole demeanor had changed! She actually stayed the whole shift and was pain-free. The night manager came to me and thanked me for taking the time to work with her knowing that I did have my reasons not to. But my reason to work with her changed instantly after I felt her energy change when she was behind me in the doctors area. That small shift in energy from negative to positive was how I had found the energy to heal... Both of us.

CHAPTER SIX

Tools: Right Words, Right Tone, Right?

Right Words, Right Tone

The Verbal Dance

Verbal Medicine™ is about effective communication using verbal and nonverbal language. This is an active skill where the dialogue changes instantly and the tempo can increase or slow down depending on the circumstances at the time of engagement.

Challenges and opportunities present themselves continuously to enable effective communication and to move a person from one state to another. The state of being out of control during an emergency that all patients find themselves in to a state of control in responding to that emergency.

That's the state healthcare workers are in. Most of the time there's a smooth transition, however there are times when it's not. Verbal Medicine™ gives you the skills to be able to move that "out of control" patient to a place where care can be provided.

Here is a great example of that:

(As related by Roger)

One evening I was working in the emergency department and one of the young charge nurses came up to me and asked if I could help with an "out of control" patient who is breathing rapidly and not responding to staff requests to slow down. I instantly said no, the staff that's caring for the patient need to use their skills to calm him down. The devil on my left shoulder made me say it and as instantly as I said that, The angel on my right shoulder had a quick word in my ear and said, "Roger, don't listen to him, you need to show them so they will know in the future." How could I refuse?

As I walked over to the room where this patient was and way before I got in the room, I could hear the antics going on inside. As I got closer and was met by one of our young male nurses (nurse Z) who had triaged the patient upon his arrival to the emergency department, he stated that the patient was in a state of panic and breathing rapidly and for 15 minutes he had been working with him in the triage room to get him to control his breathing and slow down his respiratory rate to no avail. Further more, the other nurse (nurse X) who is now taking care of the patient was also one of our young male nurses and he was trying desperately to get him to slow down his respiratory rate as well. Now, these are two great male nurses (X and Z) who work trauma and know their shit. Normally, they are great communicators but, I saw the panic in there eyes and the frustration of not being able to convince this patient to slow down his breathing. He's just not listening nor responding to them.

So now I walk into the room and I see the patient for the first time, a young Hispanic male in his 20s sitting upright in bed. He has a non-rebreather mask on to give him supplemental oxygen and he has a frothy substance coming from his mouth. His eyes are wide open and he has a fixed gaze. His respiratory rate is in the 40s! He is shirtless and I noticed various tattoos all over his body and some on his face. These are prison tattoos. I've seen tens of thousands of tattoos in my life and I'm quite familiar with prison tattoos. All the time, my two male colleagues are continually asking him to slow down his respiration rate. One of our young doctors steps into the room, Dr. G, Who looks at me and I motioned him with my hand to go away for five minutes, which he instantly did. He happily left me to work with this patient. The level of anxiety was high in the room, my two male nurses were feeding off the patient and the patient was feeding off of them.

First job, size up the situation. I have a young male Hispanic patient not responding to staff. A former prison inmate who was informing us all this by displaying his tattoos. These tattoos are all over his body including his face, once again he's telling us something about himself, he's a nonconformist. He will not do it your way. He will do it his way. We call that oppositional. Meaning, what I ask of him, he's going to do the complete opposite. Brilliant! I can work with that!

Now I know where I stand and what I need to do. So I began. I got down to his level and put my face close to his and began to break his current state.

"You're doing a great job!" I say, "Keep breathing fast, in fact I want you to breathe faster. Come on, you can do better than that! I want you to breathe faster than that!" I continued, "Because when you do, sooner or later, you're going to pass out. That's when I'll take over... that's when your mine"

His body jerked and he recoiled back from me. The two male nurses in the room also stopped in their tracks and had a puzzled look. You know that "WTF" look of astonishment.

"Yeah..." I continued, "When you pass out you will have no control of your breathing. I'm going to have to control it for you." His body jerked again and I moved away from him and pulled out a towel from a cabinet. I pull off the non rebreather mask and I wipe away the froth from his mouth that had been building up on his face. At the same time, I put my hand on his shoulder and I started to tap in a rhythmic pace matching his breathing at first and then slowing down my tapping. All the time I am talking to him at first fast and as the rhythm of my tapping slowed down so did my tone and speed, Eventually, I got to the point of asking him to allow us to take care of him, I'm occupying his mind while his body is receiving nonverbal communication by the tapping of my hand. Within three minutes I get him to the point where he calls me "Vato." Now I don't know much Spanish, but I knew what that meant from living in San Diego, which informally means guy or dude. I tell him last time I heard that was from my good Mexican friends in California. Now I'm building rapport. I keep tapping but the pace has slowed considerably down, and guess what, so has his breathing, he's matching his breathing to my tapping subconsciously. He's doing this because he is in control, there was no way he was going to have me be in control when he passed out, his subconscious mind would not allow that. he became calm and began talking to the nurses in the room, had just broken up with his girlfriend and he was very upset, that's when the doctor walked in, and I made my exit.

I was joined by the two nurses X and Z, Who asked me what the hell had just happened in there. How was I able to do that, that is, take him from an out-of-control state into a more receptive state within five minutes. I informed my two colleagues that Red flags were being thrown everywhere, the patient was telling us about himself and that they were not picking up on all of the clues he was leaving.

The fact that Nurses X and Z we're both close to 6 foot and each of them had gray scrubs on, possibly reminded him of being in prison. Remember, under stress the mind fills in the blanks with what it's familiar with. Wiping the froth from his mouth before he gave up control of his breathing convinced him subconsciously I was there to take care of him, before he had to give me something, which for him was compliance. These little things culminated in creating a positive change in everyone's lives. The person receiving the care, and more importantly the caregivers that provide that care. Ole`.

CHAPTER SEVEN

Tools: Compliance and Conditioning

Compliance and Conditioning

During the whole span of our lives each of us are subjects of ongoing conditioning and compliance. It starts at birth and only ends when we die. Most humans are creatures of habit or conditioning, if you will, and that also applies to compliance. Most of us follow the rules and like to get along with others without conflict. For instance, everyone knows to pull over to the side of the road to let a fire truck or ambulance pass when lights and sirens are going. That's complex, here's something more simple, pointing to a chair when someone needs to sit down without a single word being spoken. How about extending out a hand when greeting a person to shake hands?

Compliance and conditioning are used to full advantage in hypnosis to move a person from one state to another. From the waking state to the trance state. Sales people also take full advantage of life long conditioning and compliance knowing that when they get customers saying yes 4-5 times in a row to a series of questions related to the customers needs and wants, they have a higher chance of closing the deal when they ask for the sale.

Verbal Medicine™ also takes advantage of the in-depth knowledge pertaining to conditioning and compliance from the hypnosis and NLP perspective and combines it with the nursing process to enable the patient to get what they truly need to successfully heal. Verbal Medicine™ changes patients perceptions both physically and emotionally . Verbal Medicine™ is unique in that it builds on small successes to accumulate into Gigantic results. Verbal Medicine™ instills resilience and identifies inner resources in patients who use their "access point" to set themselves up for future success in every area of their life.

Where as most Hypnotists use compliance activities such as the "lemon test" and "magic fingers" to build up trust and belief that something MIGHT happen, The Patient Whisperers use every day nursing processes and tasks to elicit and identify signs of compliance, based on life long conditioning during healthcare interactions to build upon the expectation of care that something WILL happen.

Using the tenants of Verbal Medicine™, we have developed two techniques of relaxation inductions using these processes and the every day tools of the trade most healthcare workers have available at the bedside. They have been very powerful for identifying compliance and have been used to relax many patients. However, you don't need to be a healthcare worker to use them and they are available for use with anyone in any situation with a little practice. (See the "Gifts" chapter)

"Compliance is the key to healing."

To clarify the above statement, compliance of the patient is the key to their healing. If there is no compliance, the patient will not follow the plan of care and the path of recovery.

Healthcare professionals have two tools available that they UNDER use every single day to test for compliance. The stethoscope and the blood pressure cuff. And here's why, everyone from a child to an adult knows that the stethoscope is used for listening to the lungs and they will be asked to take a deep breath, Right? So, everyone is conditioned and will comply with taking a deep breath when this equipment is being used. With additional training, one can induce relaxation and even lead the subject into a deep trance!

The blood pressure cuff is used in a similar fashion. When a subject is told a blood pressure needs to be taken, they will automatically raise the arm closest to you even though you did not instruct them to do so because they are conditioned to do that. That is compliance. In fact, if they raised the arm farthest away, it would signify an oppositional personality or a control issue (unless they have a medical condition or injury in the near side arm.) Then the sensation of the pressure to the arm when the cuff is inflated is used to elicit relaxation as the cuff begins to deflate, it's a reproducible physical reaction which we combine with suggestions to induce relaxation and, with training, a deep trance.

Transformer Kid

(As related by Marc)

Early in our career, I had a 7 year old boy who came in for diffuse abdominal pain. Nothing in particular appeared painful and the boy did not appear to be in much distress. The doctor, after examining the boy, decided that he needed blood work and an IV. At that point, his father pulled me aside to inform me that the child is very needle phobic and just recently had to be held down by most of the staff at the pediatricians office to get a shot. He mentioned, it did not go well! So, I took this challenge and walked back into the room. I sat down next to the boy and began having a conversation about what his favorite things were. And the first thing he said was he loved Transformers! Now, I have a 24 -year-old daughter and know absolutely nothing about what a Transformer was! (Apparently it was a popular robot) And that was a good thing! Because I needed him to explain what the heck a Transformer was. So he proceeded to tell me that they were alien robots that were able to transform themselves into cars and trucks. To which I replied, "that's awesome! Who is your favorite one?" The reason I asked this question was because the best way to get someone (especially kids) into a deep trance is to get them deep into the details whatever it is they are passionate about. In this case, I wanted to know everything about his favorite transformer. He told me excitedly that it was Optimus Prime. And now here is the key detail… I began to ask him to describe Optimus Prime and when he was deeper into the details, I then asked him to tell me which part began to transform first! BINGO! I could see in his eyes, as they glossed over, that he was so deep into the transformer world that he was completely in trance! Now, all the while I had been tapping on his arm in the spot that I intended to start the IV in. The rhythmic tapping while going into trance created an anchor that would allow me to bring him back into trance deeper and deeper each time. As a matter of fact, I had broke state and brought him out of trance after he had described what Optimus Prime looked like and before I asked him which part transformed first. This allowed me to fractionate him and bring him back into trance deeper before starting the IV. So, while he was describing which part transformed first I began to stick the needle in his arm. Now, I am very good at IVs and I pride myself on getting the IV on the first time. I am known as an IV sniper! When there is a difficult IV, I am the one they call! So, what do you think happened with this needle phobic seven-year-old boy? I missed! Yes, I... missed! Now, I am thinking to myself, "What in the hell am I going to do now! I just blew my best chance at getting this kid to cooperate!" So I bring him back out of trance and tell him that he did an excellent job! And that unfortunately it didn't work and I would need to do it again if that was okay with him. Surprisingly, he acted as if it was no big deal and I think really just wanted to get back to telling me about the Transformers! So I gathered more gear and headed to the other side of the bed. He quickly shifted over to give me room to put my stuff down and put his arm out, ready to get back to his story! So again, tap tap tap and a nice healing breath, (which I had taught him in the beginning) and he was ready to tell me more about the Transformers! This time I asked him about his favorite character's arch nemesis to which he began to describe Megatron who was the leader and warlord of the Decepticons in vivid detail right down to his red glowing eyes! Again, I've got him! He is back into trance deeper than before! Now, I should point out a lot of kids do not close their eyes when going into trance like an adult and that's okay! At first, it kind of freaked us out and we thought we were unable to work with kids! But this case helped prove us wrong! It worked out very well and even though he didn't have his eyes closed, he was unfocused and deep into trance with his eyes open! So, while he was deep into trance I started the second attempt at the IV. Would you believe that as I stuck the needle in is vein blew up like a balloon! I immediately stopped and again thought to myself, "He is NEVER going to let me do this a third time! But, it won't hurt to ask!" As soon as I brought him out of trance and told him that that one did not work either, he immediately pointed to the other arm and suggested that I try this one! I was a little surprised but immediately moved to the other side of the bed and set up since he was very eager to get back to his story! Thankfully, a few taps, a breath, and a successful IV and blood draw later, he got to finish his story! Now, as soon as I brought him out of trance I gave him the most important post hypnotic suggestion he will ever get... I told him that he could do this anytime he went to a doctors office, hospital, medical office, dental office, or anywhere that he needed to get a needle stick because he did it so well and now knows how to do it even better each and every time because he has the power. He was all smiles and gave me a high five! His father was dumbfounded and could not believe what he had just witnessed! He was very thankful that I took the time to do that for his son.

CHAPTER EIGHT

Tools: Matching and Mirroring

Matching and Mirroring.

Matching and Mirroring is another communication skill that establishes trust and builds rapport. Verbal Medicine™ uses subtle techniques of matching and mirroring to gain compliance and de-escalate "out of control" patients. The basis of matching and mirroring is to speak subconsciously to another person using body movements and gestures that mimic those of the person you're talking too. The subconscious mind is literal, and when ones behaviors and gestures are matched by another person (subtlety, as to not appear to mock them), it suggests to the brain that they are both similar, they are alike, as if they are from the same tribe (the primitive brain still links us together this way) and subconsciously focuses on the words that bond them together. It fills in the blanks and most often it comes to the conclusion that they are congruent with each other, thereby making the other person receptive to the senders suggestions. Sounds simple enough but be warned, if matching and mirroring is blatant and not subtle, it looks as if you are making fun of the other person resulting in broken rapport and mistrust! Here is a fun exercise when you are out. Watch different groups or couples and see if you can identify which ones are in rapport by looking for signs of matching and mirroring. Look for things such as similarly crossed arms or legs, angles of bodies leaning toward or away, eating or drinking at the same time, etc. then play with it with your family or friends when you go out somewhere! When you have them in rapport, see if you can get them to follow your lead by changing positions or see if they eat or drink when you do! Have fun with it! (Tip: Don't tell them what you're doing or it will ruin the experiment!)

The Matriarch

(Excerpt from our lecture)

Marc Sacco: Building rapport, matching, mirroring, pacing. We're all familiar with matching, mirroring, and pacing. But you probably aren't familiar with the technique I used or the situation that I had to use it in. But it works tremendously well when done properly. So this was "The Angry Family." The Angry Family was probably Eastern European. So they were very abrupt. This older gentleman was the patriarch of the family and he was not feeling well. He had some belly pain. He was not feeling good at all. We're a very busy ER and they had been there..probably two to three hours, before they would be seen, before we could get stuff done. We were very busy that night. So I had four room assignments and he was my fourth patient. I'm working my way down the line. I had a difficult and time-consuming procedure called – a Port-a-cath access.

I was accessing a port – so that's a sterile procedure. You have to take the time. It's not like starting an IV where you can put it in and move on. So, all four of my patients happen to need access of their Port-a-Caths! So I'm going through and I'm doing them– I get the first and second one done no problem. The third one, I get it in and it doesn't flow. So I de-access it and start again. So now I've done four Port-a-Caths (on three patients) and I've got this fifth one and they've been waiting and waiting. They're getting all the more anxious (angry) and there's no time for me to go back in and say, "Hey, I'm going to be there soon." I saw them when they first came in and I had said I was going to be there as quickly as I can but that I had all these procedures to do before I could get to them.

They knew I was busy. But they didn't think it was going to be this long. They had already been in the waiting room for a couple of hours before getting into a room so they're getting more agitated. I finish the second Port-a-Cath attempt and I get it in no problem. I go out of the room and I hear a little bit of grumbling in the next room and the doctor comes out and says, "Can you get the CAT scan drinks?" I said, "Yes, that's where I'm coming to next."

So I go out to the med room and I'm like a bartender getting ready to mix these two big drinks, the lemonade and the Gastrografin which is a radiographic dye – and I'm mixing them up and getting ready and trying to grab the next Port-a-Cath kit. I'm getting all my stuff and one of the nurses comes rushing into the med room. He says, "Man, don't go into room four. They are pissed. They are cursing and yelling at everybody going by!" Now, I wasn't in that great of a rapport building mood to begin with. So I was a little frustrated and I said, "Well, I will take care of this." I've got my CAT scan drinks in both hands. I've got my Port-a-Cath pack all under my arm and I go rushing in.

I come into the door and they're all standing except the patient and they're angry and they're yelling and the matriarch of the family, has a very Eastern European accent and she flailing her arms around in a very angular pattern as she yells and this is the first thing I see when I get into the door! So, I've got both glasses in my hands and she's looking at me and she's screaming at me. She's is yelling, "I don't know what's going on around here! But he needs some help! And no one seems to give a DAMN!" Swinging her arms up and down and I'm thinking to myself, "Matching and mirroring? This is going to really get messy. There is no way I can do this with my hands full!"

So, I quickly put the drinks and the kit down and I had to – at this moment, put my career on the line. I said to myself, "If I'm going to do this, I'm going to have to commit 100 percent, 100 percent or its not going to work! I'm going to have to match and mirror her and pace her back down. If it doesn't work, I'm probably going to get fired." This is a defining moment for me. So I start.

I match her tone, pace and volume and yell back, "I understand! I'm upset too! I've been very busy over here, (I begin to slow down the pace, soften the tone, and change my body language) but I want to help you. I want to help him and I'm here to start that Port-a-Cath and I've got these drinks and we're going to do the best thing for you, if you will allow me. She calmed down. She matched and mirrored me immediately and was in agreement. The son on the other hand was still upset. I had been totally focused on her but now had to change focus to him. He starts yelling and cursing at me, "Well, I don't want you eff-ing touching my dad and I want a new nurse and I..." I had to do the same thing and fast... So I yelled back (purposely finishing his sentence using a pattern interrupt) with, "...I agree! It has been bad and I'm sorry and I want to be here to help him, (again slowing the pace, softening the tone, and changing the body language) I continued, "... if you will allow me to. I'm here for you. I'm going to dedicate getting this taken care of. And I want to thank you for opportunity to help." That was it. From then on until they left (when the patient was admitted) they were pleasant, accommodating and understanding. I walked them out after he was admitted. When they left, I escorted them out the four doors to the waiting room and he shook my hand six times along the way! And as I walked the son out and he was shaking my hand he said, "Thank you so much for listening to me and caring for my father," At that point (the last door) I thought he was going to hug me! It really was phenomenal. They were so grateful.

Now the funny thing is we all like watching train wrecks. We can't help it, right? Well, nurses are even more like that. Out in the nurse's station, you could see like eight different people crammed inside looking into the room, the whole time, behind me. They were waiting for this verbal massacre, this bloody thing to happen. They were amazed, because they saw this whole thing transform before their eyes.

Nobody could talk to the "Angry Family" because when I was mixing drinks, they were yelling at them and there was no communication, because they couldn't talk the same language and their intent was not right. They were on different planes. We see that all the time. Nurses go in, "I'm sorry, but I'm busy and we're…blah, blah, blah…" – they can't hear that. The staff is talking here (points down low) and they're (the patients) talking a different language and they're up here (points up high).

Roger Woods: It was remarkable. It was great.

Marc Sacco: And… I still had my job!

CHAPTER NINE

Tools: Pacing and Leading

Pacing and Leading

Pacing and leading are two factors that assist with bringing a patient from an "out of control" state into a state of healing and compliance. We have to meet the patient at the level they are currently at and skillfully bring them down to a point where they are receptive to what we are saying and compliant with what needs to be done for them. The key here is rhythm and speed. Not too fast or not too slow, being ahead just a fraction as not to leave them behind, adjusting to every reaction. They talk fast you talk faster at the beginning and then slow down, and when you slow down, they will come with you and will be more receptive to what you are saying.

(Excerpt from our lecture...)

Roger Woods: To the Naked Dorm Guy!

Marc Sacco: Naked Dorm Guy. I was waiting for that part. So, Naked Dorm Guy. We have a college right near the hospital and they got a call for a naked guy running through the dorms, completely butt-ass naked and actually they found him in the women's locker room showers. So it took 10 officers to get him into the ambulance. Thankfully, they had gotten him dressed at that point. It took them an hour and a half to get him coaxed into the ambulance. You now have your two paramedics, a police officer and a patient in the back of the ambulance and they come to the ER.

They back up into the ambulance bay and then we're waiting. Fifteen minutes goes by and there's still no patient, still nobody comes out of the ambulance. So I go out and I see there's a stretcher out there with the four-point restraints hanging on it, sitting outside the ambulance. There are four security guards, five police officers and two paramedics and they were all talking to this guy, trying to get him to come in. He's kind of yelling his speech. He's not "angry" yelling, just oppositional. So anytime they said something like, "Hey, my lieutenant needs me to get back to the station. Can you just come into the hospital? I got paperwork to do." He would respond, "No, no, no!" First thing, "No, no, no! I don't want to do that. I want to go home. No, no, no! I want out." So he was saying specific things. I was sitting back. I'm watching another 15 minutes go by. It's about 30 minutes total and I'm kind of enjoying it but I was actually just getting some more information. They were putting the gloves on just getting ready to yank this guy out.

Now that was my cue! I don't want any injuries to the patient, injuries to the security, or injuries to the police officers. Everybody is going to have some sort of injury in trying to drag this guy out of an ambulance. So I said, "Hold on. Let me do this." I walk up and I introduce myself to him. He's still sitting on the bench seat in the ambulance and I tell him who I am, that I'm a nurse and I just start engaging some talk with him.

Basically I used some NLP type languaging where I said, "You're here and this is a one-way street. The only way to move forward ..." That's the other thing... I wanted to give him that activity of moving forward. So I continued, "...the only way to move forward and get out and go home is to get out of the ambulance and walk forward." Notice that I was using a blend of his words (get out, go home) and my intentions (move forward) to create sentences that he could comprehend and felt like something he would have thought up on his own!

And he says, "OK' and begins to get out of the ambulance! Everybody is looking around. They're getting ready because they've got the bed with the four points nearby. They're thinking, OK, maybe he's just going to bolt after he gets out. So they were getting ready. But he gets out and moves forward toward the doors.

I continued, "We're going to move forward. We're going to go through these doors." And of course he said, "No, no, no!" Now, I already know he is oppositional and I have about five sets of doors to get through. So we get to the first one and I said,

"Yeah, so we're going to go in through here and go into that room." He again said, "No, no, no! I don't want to. I want to go home." I continued without missing a beat, "Great, because this is a one-way street and the only way to get out and go home is to go forward!" Now, I started changing those three sentences a little bit each time while using these words "forward, out and home." I just started using those three words in sentences every time he said no and it worked every single time.

"Oh, OK." He said and walked through the set of doors and we get to another door. "OK, we're going to go in this one." "No, no, no!", I use more sentences with… "Forward, out, home." And we go through another door. We're getting all the way through the five doors into the little room and the security guards come in with the gown and pants and socks because every behavioral care patient has to get completely naked and put a gown on for safety. We've had a nurse friend of ours shot in the chest so we're very picky about that kind of thing. So security guard comes in and says, "Hey, you have to get all your clothes off and put this gown." "No, no, no! Not going to do it." So, again, "forward, out, home," three variations of the sentences. He Strips butt naked and gets his gown on without any help. The Doctor comes in and he hasn't built any rapport whatsoever and says, "Hey, what's going on?" Of course he answers, "No, I just want to go home. I want to get out of here. I want to move forward." Notice he changed what he said? He started saying he wanted to move forward! That was a big clue to me but not this doctor! The doctor didn't bother to take the time to listen to what was said nor did he wait for any information from me as to what progress I had made! The doctor replied, "You're not going anywhere." (Pointing to me) "Medicate him." And he walked out. So now we are potentially going to have to wrestle him down, put him in four-point restraints, get two needles, give him two different shots (commonly referred to as a "B-52"). This could be a nightmare. Instead, I said, "Hey, I've got a great idea! In order to move forward through this, the doctor needs to give you some medication to get you home eventually. You can do it one of two ways. One way, the easy way is if you just lay on the stretcher, let them put those restraints on, so you're safe, we're safe and we can give you the medication or you can allow them to assist you into the bed and put these four-point restraints on. We can hold you down and it's not as good a way. If you want to really move forward in this and get out of here, I suggest you just lay on the bed."

He immediately agreed, "OK." And he literally got on the bed, put his arms and his legs out into the restraints himself and security clicked him in. I gave him the shots. No wrestling, no nothing. Done. Just like that. That was Naked Dorm Guy!

CHAPTER TEN

Professionalism: See it, Act it, Be it

BODY TALK
See it, Act it, Be it.

Verbal Medicine™ is more than just using words, it takes advantage of using the other 80% of effective communication, and that is, body language. You see, we constantly use our bodies to communicate much more than we do our words. And when our words and body language are incongruent (out of balance), the communication is in discourse, and the message is lost. Our bodies always subconsciously communicate what we are deeply thinking automatically to the outside world. A skillful practitioner is able to decipher the occult code and make sense of it consciously instead of just reacting from a subconscious level. That old saying "you wear your heart on your sleeve", is very true except it's not just one sleeve, it's all over your body! The clothes and jewelry you wear, the way you walk, talk, move and breathe. It's your posture, positioning, and stance. It's also in the tone of your voice, the cadence, pitch and speed of delivery in your voice (see other chapters). And what is just as important, the intent of the message being sent are all factors that go into effective communication.

The first impression is the most important tool one can control, and the first impression is mostly visual. We see first from a distance and make snap decisions then we continue to look for more clues in our evaluation, on a subconscious level, until we have made decision on how we feel about the situation. That is our "Gut Feeling".

Have you ever instantly taken a dislike to someone? You have a "feeling" that you just cannot explain or put your finger on. Well that is your subconscious mind at work, it's filling in the blanks without any effort from you. It has a habit of creating little movies with little bits of information that you begin to react too. We all do it, and the reactions can be profound whether you are daydreaming, having a fantasy, or worse, a nightmare.

So first impressions are extremely important if you want to establish trust and success.

We use six words with every person we work with to challenge and change their perception.

SEE IT, ACT IT, BE IT.

These six simple words are very powerful in changing a persons perception of self and confidence.

We encourage our clients and patients to see themselves successful in the future. What will it look like? What will it feel like when they have that success? What will it do for them? We then instill how their image of success would act by presenting types of activity and behaviors that will be associated with that image. We then tell them to start acting now just as that image will act in the future with the success they want. The final part of the change is that they begin to be the mirror image they want to be right now by owning the behavior and being that vision of success right now, because....if you... SEE IT you can ACT IT and if you ACT IT you can BE IT... Right!

(As related by Roger) This brings me to a wonderful story with a young resident doctor I had the pleasure of interacting with. Actually it was a forced interaction by me, and here is why.

Many weeks I had followed this particular medical resident into "my" patients rooms after he had spoken to them about being admitted to the hospital for care. Each time I asked the patient what the Doctor had asked, they were always surprised that the person they had spoken too was indeed a "Doctor", and more importantly that he was going to be the one taking care of them during their stay in the hospital. His first impression had left a very negative one. This was because of a couple of factors, firstly he dressed like a sack of... "potatoes", and thats putting it mildly. You see, he didn't look the part of a medically trained professional , he had enormous clump of unkept hair that I'm sure there were birds nesting in it, he had a hippie like beard, not groomed and out of control all over his face, he was constantly wearing wrinkled scrubs with (what I hope were only food) stains on the front, his white coat had a big ink stain on the pocket and was fraying on both of the elbows, and I would bet good money it had never seen the inside of a washing machine. His bedroom floor... yes, a washing machine... not so much. So, not only did he not look the part, he didn't believe he was the part. He still believed his exterior image was acceptable by acting and dressing as he did when he was a struggling medical student, after all he had lived with this mental image for the past 5 years. So, by not "looking" the part and not "acting" the part, there was no way he could BE the part. Not only did he believe he was the medical student and not the Doctor subconsciously with his choice of attire and attitude, but guess what, everyone he came in contact with also believed he wasn't the Doctor.

His verbal language and his body language where not congruent and therefore he was sending a mixed message, subconsciously and unintentionally.

This continued day after day until I intervened. I liked this resident, he was always polite, intelligent and was quite funny to interact with. Because I had great rapport with him, I knew I would have an opportunity to help him with what I had seen and what "our" patients had experienced with their interaction with him.

Often patients ask if I'm the Doctor, for various reasons due to stereotyping and conditioning over a lifetime. First, I am male and most doctors are male. Second, I don't dress like the typical nurse in scrubs, in fact only 50% of the time do I wear a scrub top, however I always wear a collared shirt and I always have either my name embroidered on it or a name tag on it. I put my name on my product, and my product is me. I wear pants and I very rarely wear sneakers. I dress and look the part of someone who is confident, clean and well-kept, my clothes are always ironed prior to wear and I project an image of professionalism.

I practice what I preach, I model good behavior, and so I come from a position of authority when I talk about this to students and coworkers.

I began our conversation with my intent, which was feedback not criticism. Feedback comes from a place of love and not that of malice, my feedback is a gift, I'm choosing to give a gift of feedback, and one can do what they want with it, just know it comes from a place of love. So knowing this helps to take the sting out of what is about to be said, right? Because I know the truth sometimes can hurt, right? It hurts to hear it and it hurts to say it... right?

So I told him, "Do you realize that almost every time I follow you into "our" patients room, they all say the same thing after you leave the room? Most cannot believe you are the Doctor because of how you look. It's not about what you know, it's about how you look, and how you carry yourself, and most patients are conditioned that doctors dress a certain way, it's a crucial part of the expectancy of care that doctors and nurses provide. Right? And if "OUR" patients do not believe that you look and act like a doctor, then how will they believe in the plan of care that you want them to follow, how you look and how you carry yourself has a great influence over the patients we are going to provide care for. Right?"

(Here's a little NLP technique), every time I make a statement, I get agreement by using the word 'right' immediately after stating it, right? And when the receiver of that statement says either right or yes, the subconscious mind picks that up as a suggestion. Right? And when you get agreement, you can start to change perception which results in a different response. Right?

Over the last five years, we have found great results start by changing perceptions incrementally at first. It's the domino effect were looking for. Change one small thing and that will change another and then another and it goes on culminating with a profound change in perception in how the subject thinks and more importantly how they react.

So, I talked to him about how I prepare every morning and the reason why, I explained to him how I need to change the state of our patients from being the subject of a condition or diagnosis. The goal is to allow them to follow a path of recovery and using this time to show that they do have inner resources to help with all aspects of their life and not just in the health of their bodies, but also with the health of their minds. Right? (see how easy it is, right?)

"Our" conversation took no more than 10 minutes, and yes, I did all the talking, suggesting, modeling, basically what we call in traditional Hypnosis as "waking hypnosis".

Some weeks passed and I had forgotten about our encounter until out of the corner of my eye I noticed an unfamiliar person walking down the hallway. From a distance, I couldn't make out who it was but the person was dressed in a shirt and tie with pressed trousers and a freshly pressed clean white lab coat. His face was clean shaven, tight haircut and a swagger to his walk. As he came closer, I finally realized who this person was.....yep, that young Doctor I had the encounter with some weeks earlier. As he came closer he began to smile and put out his hand to shake mine and as we did, he began to discuss his transformation and the reaction he had been receiving in return.

Because of his transformation, he had noticed people reacted by treating him differently and even seek out his opinion on medical matters! After all, he was very intelligent and had worked hard to gain the knowledge. However, people previously only focused on what they saw, not what he knew. Now the tables had turned, he looked like a Doctor and the more he began to act like the Doctor, he suddenly was treated like THE DOCTOR. Now they came to him for his wisdom, which is the application of knowledge. And what had he learned? You have to see you are the Doctor and act like the Doctor, to be the Doctor. Right? (There I go again)

CHAPTER ELEVEN
Resources and Training

The National Guild of Hypnotists, Inc (NGH)

Established in 1950, the Guild has grown to over 20,000 members, with over 100 local chapters in 89 different countries. A growing percentage of our members have academic credentials in other fields, including medicine, psychology, counseling and nursing.

The National Guild of Hypnotists[12] has been acknowledged, even by other professional hypnotism groups, as the number one association in the field. We invite you to share in the prestige and recognition membership brings, by joining the nation's premier hypnosis organization.

Neuro Linguistic Programming (NLP)

While there certainly are several reputable resources for training and information about NLP we only endorse the ones we have had personal associations with. First and foremost is Dr. Matt James at NLP.com and The Empowerment Partnership[13]. We trained directly with him and it was a life changing event (Twice!!) We highly recommend training with him if you get the chance and his entry level training is very cost effective (at this writing it is under $200 for a 4 day basic training event)

Dr. William Horton[14] is a valued member of the NGH and well regarded instructor in NGH & NLP.

Dr. Richard Bandler[15], is the Co-Founder of the field of Neuro-Linguistic Programming. A distinguished visitor to Menninger's Foundation, a Keynote Speaker for many Associations and Foundations.

Verbal Medicine™

One day Verbal Medicine™ seminars are held throughout the year at various venues in the United States and Canada and can be found at our website. The Patient Whisperers™ are available to teach seminars internationally and can be contacted through the website or the email address in the front of the book.

Lectures are held at many of the national conventions for hypnosis and nursing as well as many institutions and universities. The Patient Whisperers™ are also available for lecturing internationally and can be contacted through the website or the email address in the front of the book.

CRNH™

The Certified Registered Nurse Hypnotist (CRNH™) certification[16] is recognized as the premiere course for all disciplines of nursing and empowers nurses with the knowledge and hands on skills to provide expert care to patients across a wide spectrum of care and measures the attainment of a defined body of nursing knowledge pertinent to this specialty.

Developed by The Patient Whisperers™ over 4 years and over 25,000 patients, to give all Registered Nurses the training and understanding to apply hypnosis, NLP and Verbal Medicine™ to patient care in all aspects of nursing. Usually taught in conjunction with a 100 hour NGH certified hypnosis course, it can also be taken as a post certification 3 day intensive workshop.

Conventions and Additional Trainings

Here is a small list of conventions and trainings we recommend if you would like to learn more about Hypnosis, NLP and Verbal Medicine™.

National & International Conventions

NGH, Marlborough, MA in August

HypnothoughtsLive, Las Vegas, in August

IMDHA, Daytona, FL in May

Trainings

The Patient Whisperers

Ron Eslinger

The Elmann's

Ines Simpson

Mike Mandel

Melissa Tiers

Dr. Matt James

Mark Schwimmer

Joanna Cameron

Jason Linett

Roy Hunter

CHAPTER TWELVE

The Gifts

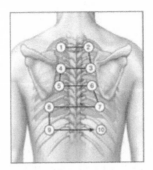

The Stethoscope Relaxation Induction™

1. Invoke a memory. Use visual stimuli.

"You remember a time when you went to a doctors office, a hospital, or any medical facility, and the doctor or the nurse listened to your lungs, right? " *(show client the stethoscope)*

2. Invoke an emotion and feeling.

"You remember how that felt , right? Well, I want you to remember what that was like and in a moment we are going to do that again…"

3. Invoke a sensation. Use Kinesthetic stimuli. Use anchoring.

Is it OK with you if I place my hand on your shoulder like this? *(Place one hand on the near shoulder and the head of the stethoscope on position 1. During each breath, you will tap the shoulder rhythmically to mimic a heartbeat continually thereby anchoring it into this state of relaxation)* " Normally, they would place the stethoscope here and ask you to take a nice deep relaxing breath in through your nose, hold it...and let it out slowly through your mouth. That's right, good... Now close your eyes, and do it again. *(change to position 2)* In through the nose, hold it, and out through the mouth slowly. that's right, and as you breathe out, allow your head to come forward...that's right, allow it to come forward and as it comes forward, allow yourself to go straight down into a wonderful state of relaxation. That's right. *(change to position 5)* Again, deep breath in through the nose, hold it, and out slowly relaxing deeper and deeper... just focus now as your head goes down further and further and gets heavier and heavier, you can go down deeper and deeper... *(change to position 6)* breathe in......hold.....breathe out and just let it all go down, deeper and deeper... *(put aside stethoscope and put other hand on back of the neck and gently sway client side to side while continuing to tap out a heartbeat rhythm on the shoulder)* breathe and go deeper.... that's right, notice how relaxed you are....breathe and go deeper...

4.   **Gentle fractionation. Re-emerge the client. Invoke anchor to induce.**

And on the count of three you will open your eyes. One, getting ready to come back into the room. Two, take a nice big deep breath in. Three, open your eyes feeling absolutely wonderful and notice how relaxed you are. That's great.... now *(start tapping on the shoulder again)* I want you to breathe and relax, breathe and relax, that's right, breathe.....and....relax...going deeper and deeper into that wonderful relaxing state you enjoyed a moment ago...

5. **Suggestions and trance work.**

(Insert whatever your client needs here...)

6. **Re-emerge client.**

And on the count of three you will open your eyes. One, getting ready to come back into the room. Two, take a nice big deep breath in. Three, open your eyes feeling absolutely wonderful and notice how relaxed you are. That's right....

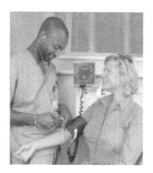

The BP Cuff Relaxation Induction™

1. Invoke a memory. Use visual stimuli.

"You remember a time when you went to a doctors office, a hospital, or any medical facility, and the doctor or the nurse took your blood pressure, right? " *(Show client the stethoscope and/or BP Cuff)*

2. **Invoke an emotion and feeling.**

"You remember how that felt, right? Well, I want you to remember what that was like and in a moment we are going to do that again..."

3. **Invoke a sensation. Use Kinesthetic stimuli. Use anchoring.**

**"Now, let's get ready to take a blood pressure" *(Don't say anymore*
words and wait for the client to move their arm into the horizontal
position, as this shows they are compliant. When the

arm moves, place the blood pressure cuff on the arm and give it a slight squeeze.) "That's right...now I'm going to inflate the cuff but not too tight on THIS arm." *(Inflate the blood pressure cuff to a comfortable but tight pressure of no more than 80mmHg**.)* "Close your eyes and focus your attention on the sensation of the blood pressure cuff on THAT arm." *(Dissociating the arm being used)* "In a moment, I will release that pressure in the cuff..... slowly, and when you notice that pressure decreasing... notice how good it feels as the tension releases and the muscles relax. Then send that sensation to the whole arm, all right?" *(Release the pressure anchoring it to a state of relaxation.)* "That felt good, right? Good... Now, keep your eyes closed and we will do it again. This time send that sensation of release and relaxation down both arms and double the sensation." *(Re-inflate the cuff. Release the pressure a little slower than before.)* "Now, allow that sensation of release and relaxation to double and move right now, down both arms, that's right, relaxing, releasing, releasing, relaxing, doubling that sensation, that's right"........."Keep your eyes closed now". "That's right, now take a deep breath, hold it.....and let it out slowly.....that's right"

"Now, you are going to do this one more time, still keeping your eyes closed, and this time send that relaxation all over your body" "That's right"

(Inflate the cuff a little more tighter this time, and deflate even longer.) "Now, imagine sending that sensation of release and relaxation all over your body now from head to toe, that's right, relaxing, releasing, relaxing, releasing, as tension releases, muscles relax, the whole of your body becoming so relaxed now ,.... so heavy,..... so loose,....thats right"

4. **Gentle fractionation. Re-emerge the client. Invoke anchor to induce.**

"In a moment I'm going to count to three, then and only then on the count of three you will open your eyes. One, getting ready to come back into the room. Two, take a nice big deep breath in. Three, open your eyes feeling absolutely wonderful and notice how relaxed you are. That's great...." *(Inflate the cuff a little bit or squeeze the arm and release it.)* "Now I want you to close your eyes, breathe and relax, breathe and relax, that's right, breathe.....and....relax...going deeper and deeper into that wonderful relaxing state you enjoyed a moment ago...

5. **Suggestions and trance work.**

(Insert whatever your client needs here...)

6. **Re-emerge client.**

And on the count of three you will open your eyes. One, getting ready to come back into the room. Two, take a nice big deep breath in. Three, open your eyes feeling absolutely wonderful and notice how relaxed you are. That's right...

**This induction can be done without BP cuff by either squeezing the arm or having the client tighten the arm to simulate the cuff inflating. Also, maximum pressure of 100mmHg should be used by non-medical personnel.

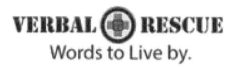

"Fall seven times, stand up eight."

— Japanese Proverb

Our mission is to help everyone survive life without burning out through easy to learn tools using self-hypnosis and Neuro Linguistic Programming (NLP) to learn to erase the negative baggage that weighs us all down and allow us all to change our perception of life to attain positive well-being. Verbal Rescue™ is the umbrella concept that covers the methods of Verbal Medicine™, Hypnosis, and NLP that can help with the overload of life that can cause burnout in work, home, social situations, and relationships.

3 Stages of Verbal Rescue

$$ER^3$$

Emotional Reception
> Identify
>
> Acknowledge
>
> Accept

Emotional Response
> Forgive
>
> Empower
>
> Plan

Emotional Reward
> Center
>
> Balance
>
> Release

Verbal Rescue Script

*(This is a sample script used for people who help others such as First Responders and Healthcare workers. The script is to be inserted in between a progressive relaxation and the emerging from a relaxation session.)

The amazing gift about our work.... is that we are placed into peoples lives.... at their time of need....

And that's when....our work is meaningful....to us.

Our work.... is deep in our lives....it's in our blood....it's the very essence of who we are....and what we are.... in the universe....

We are called to respond....and we do each and every day....

Ever so vigilant....ever so prepared.... ever so calm and confident....professional and competent....

We rush in....as others are running out.... That's what we do.... that's who we are....

Always on duty....for strangers, family and friends....

We heal and help....in so many ways....There is something that drives us.... propels us....to serve our fellow man....

And we have that power....to forgive....where others hold on to that hurt....

we make sense of it and.... use it for good....

Allowing only positive energy.... through our armor.... that protects us from the pain.... and the strain....that is part of our work....

We find the energy to heal....even at times when we have a little reserves....

Our capabilities are endless....

There is a balance in our lives.... with the giving and taking....

That's why we have passion.... in what we do....passion for what we love....passion for who we love....and let into our lives....

We bring sunshine when there is dark....warmth when there is coldness.... release....when there is stress....and comfort when there is pain....

We have a center that follows our moral compass....true north....

It leads the way to success....and happiness....

This is who we are.... this is what we do....and it cannot be done without you....

CHAPTER THIRTEEN
Summary and Conclusion

The development of Verbal Medicine™ began soon after we received training in Hypnosis and NLP, in fact it was an easy transition to merge the techniques with the nursing process which we both use every day as registered nurses working in the emergency department.

As Verbal Medicine™ developed over the years, we noticed greater change and phenomenal results in both the patients under our care, the professionals we work with, and the work we were doing personally. The work we were doing signified something totally different now. It felt different because it was different. The energy had changed and the biggest change came in the pair of us. We have talked much in this book about energy, to be precise, the energy to heal. We know we talk for all healthcare professionals when we say that constantly giving to our patients causes our energy to fade out within the first five years. What's alarming is that statistics show that nurses burn out within five years and quit working in hospitals all together in search of a less stressful work environment. And we were no different, we were burnt out in our caregiving and close to moving away from the hospital environment all together. The environment had changed, we no longer had time at the bedside to engage our patients, other duties sucked up our time at the bedside, tasks, charting, inefficiency and short staffing for getting the best of us. We were no longer nurses, we were mechanics or technicians working on and repairing widgets. We were quickly losing the "care" in our "healthcare." Truthfully, we were looking in a different direction and by the grace of God and the power of the universe, we were able to enroll in a Hypnosis certification course that instantly changed our outdated thoughts and negative thinking. It put us on a path to change the way healthcare is delivered at the bedside and more importantly, how it is perceived, not just by the healthcare professional, but by the patients receiving it.

We learned that when the delivery changes, so do the results. We found that by developing Verbal Medicine™ we, the confident, efficient, amazing professionals that most nurses are, began to drive the care in a real holistic direction, because we know what needs to be done, and that is so powerful to know. Also, patients who come to us have an expectation of care, and they yield control over to us as healthcare professionals to get that care. So, building on that resource of influence given to us by the patient, we should be engaged in a way that they follow our lead, our directions, and our suggestions using the Verbal Medicine™ communication skills. Instead we found that patients are all too often left to fill in the blank's when communication and information is withheld or not delivered at all. And when they fill in the blank's, all too often they fill it with negative information which leads to noncompliance with care, frustration directed towards the healthcare professionals, and dissatisfaction, which in the long run can be very detrimental to healthcare institutions both financially and with their reputation in the community.

As Verbal Medicine™ developed, we started to notice a big difference when we purposely changed our words when talking to patients, family members and even coworkers. In fact, we made it somewhat of a challenge to change each and everyone's negative words into positive words. Because we know what we say to ourselves our subconscious believes.

Have you ever done something wrong and called yourself an idiot, stupid, etc.? Well, the subconscious picks up on that, stores that, remembers that, and allows you to believe that. So why allow that to happen.? Why not just say positive things to yourself instead. You know, we would never ever say to a stranger all of the negative things we say about ourselves. So why do we do that? When you change this one aspect of your life, how you talk to yourself, you will notice how better life can be.

One of the biggest detrimental factors to healthcare over the last 20 years has been the one little question that is asked and even mandated to be addressed... that is the one concerning pain.

Talk about a stimulus response loop! We see it all the time. We are required to ask patients about their pain level many times during their visit and immediately when we do, believe it or not, subconsciously we have just given them a Suggestion for pain! They may have been sitting there comfortably, talking to a family member or staff member, not complaining or showing any outward signs of symptoms of being in discomfort, but immediately when you ask, they have it. It also could be a family member, asking the patient out of concern but once again subconsciously suggesting to a patient that they are in pain when they say " are you in pain" or even worse, "How much pain are you in!?"

And what's the first thing that the doctor will do? You got it, prescribe pain medication. Because it's quick, and they are mandated to treat a person's pain. Whether or not the pain is real or not, we see it as a huge problem where people are being medicated when there is no real disabling pain. There's a pill for everything, nobody has to feel anything anymore, all they need to feel is numb. Nobody takes the time to help these patients manage their discomfort. Because there is a difference between pain and discomfort. And you can change pain to discomfort. People can and do live in discomfort, but nobody has the time to change a person's perception of debilitating pain to a manageable discomfort. Until Verbal Medicine™ that is!

We change everything about that person's perception, and give them the skills to change how things feel and what it means exactly. We are empowering them to live a better life, in control of that discomfort instead of being powerless to the pain. It's all about control, they can control the intensity, they can control the duration. They can control the size and the shape using their focus and imagination. Because, as Rudyard Kipling said, "Words are the most powerful drug used by mankind," and we use them wisely to heal.

We use those same powerful words to help insert IVs or obtain labs and work with patients who are needle phobic to change the way they feel and perceive procedures as well as give them resources for the future when they need these services. Simply, we set them up for success!

We never ever say these words "poke, bee sting, stick, pinch etc." because the moment you say that,

that's exactly what they're going to feel, because we just gave them that suggestion. So with Verbal Medicine™, we allow them to feel whatever they want to feel or nothing at all! (For a great demonstration, look up The Patient Whisperers' YouTube video called, "TPW sutures using only Verbal Medicine™".) It sounds simple, and let us tell you, it is. It is remarkable what you can do just using words.

The right words that is, the words that heal.

~TPW

Endnotes

---

[1] (Grolier Electronic Publishing, Inc. 1990)

[2] http://www.nlplifetraining.com/what-is-nlp/index.html

[3] Notes on Nursing, Florence Nightingale, 1860

[4] https://harvardmagazine.com/2013/01/the-placebo-phenomenon

[5] https://harvardmagazine.com/2013/01/the-placebo-phenomenon

[6] Garland, E.L., Baker, A.K., Larsen, P. et al. J GEN INTERN MED (2017) 32: 1106. https://doi.org/10.1007/s11606-017-4116-9

[7] https://www.amazon.com/The-Worst-Is-Over-Moment/dp/1494376539/ref=sr_1_2?ie=UTF8&qid=1396471084&sr=8-2

[8] Healing Words for Trauma Victims
http://www.teachingvirtues.net

[9] Frisch, N. (May 31, 2001). "Nursing as a Context for Alternative/Complementary Modalities". Online Journal of Issues in Nursing. Vol. 6 No. 2, Manuscript 2. Available: www.nursingworld.org//MainMenuCategories/ANAMarketplace/ANAPeriodicals/OJIN/TableofContents/Volume62001 /No2May01/AlternativeComplementaryModalities.aspx

[10] https://www.jointcommission.org/assets/1/18/R3_Report_Issue_11_Pain_Assessment_8_25_17_FINAL.pdf

[11] Healthy Visions www.healthyvisions.com

[12] https://new.ngh.net

[13] http://www.empowermentpartnership.com

[14] http://www.drwillhorton.com

[15] http://www.nlplifetraining.com/richard-bandler

[16] http://www.nursehypnotist.com

Made in the USA
Monee, IL
12 July 2021